PRAISE FOR SHIFT YOUR CONFIDENCE

"My experience with Samantha Hill as a coach was enlightening and life-changing. Samantha's compassionate and intuitive coaching style and techniques helped me grow and gained the confidence I needed to proactively move forward with my personal and professional goals. She is genuine, honest, warm, empowering and endlessly encouraging. I highly recommend Coach Samantha and her coaching sessions and programs as effective mindset transformation tools."
— Tonya Griffin, Certified Life, Wellness and Career Transition Coach

"I know your book will inspire others as it has definitely impacted my life. I have seen my attitude about myself, my career, and launching my businesses shift 180 degrees. Thank you for your coaching and lively worthwhile training and encouraging me to 'Trust the Process.'"
— Debbie Whitlock, Allied Healthcare Professional Respiratory Therapist

"I have known Samantha for several years and have had the opportunity to consult with her on many projects. Samantha is a highly motivated individual who excels at opportunities that require innovation and self-motivation. The pride she takes in everything she is a part of comes through in her commitment and drive."
— Latosha Dexter, Deputy University Counsel

"I cannot wait to see this book on the shelf. There are so many real-life applications you can really appreciate about life."
— Dama Lee, Director of Dama's Little Folks Child Care Center

"So great to have reconnected with such a powerful and inspiring woman. Being a part of the Confidence for Women group brings unity. Thank you for the Empowerment and Motivation. I wish you much success."
— Emma Williams Holmes, Executive Administrative Assistant

"I would like to give my sincere thanks to Samantha Wisdom Hill for her dedication in accelerating me forward and toward my career as an Esthetician. I enrolled in her Confident Shift Program to enhance my self-care, self-esteem and to regain my power to set forth my path of becoming an entrepreneur. I now have begun my journey as CEO. Thank you and many blessings and prosperity with your book of empowering women!!"
— Leiwanna Bourroughs, Purple Orchid Skincare LLC

"After going through the program The Confident Shift, it helps to build my confidence and schedule my daily tasks to help me not to overwhelm myself."
— Keishea Hurdle, Burton Legacy, seamstress

"Coach Samantha has been so encouraging and enthusiastic about our life and future, I know the book will be phenomenal. It's a must read. You will be blessed."
— Evangelist Linda Moreno

SHIFT YOUR CONFIDENCE!

SHIFT YOUR CONFIDENCE!

A 15-Day Journey to *FIRE* Negative Self-Talk

SAMANTHA HILL

Shift Your Confidence! A 15-Day Journey to FIRE Negative Self-Talk

Copyright © 2021 by Samantha Hill

Published by INYLegacy Press
Website: https://www.confidentshift.com

ISBN (paperback): 978-1-7378320-0-3
ISBN (ebook): 978-1-7378320-1-0

Edited by Jessica Vineyard, Red Letter Editing, www.redletterediting.com
Book design by Christy Day, Constellation Book Services,
www.constellatiobookservices.com

Printed in the United States of America

First, to the head of my life whom I acknowledge in everything that I do...my Lord and Savior.

To my husband, Brian Hill, I will be forever grateful for your love and support. You truly keep me grounded and shooting for the stars.

To my Queen Sisters in my private Facebook group called Confidence for Women for encouraging me to write this book on how to FIRE negative self-talk.

CONTENTS

INTRODUCTION

"Girl, you need to write a book. Every time I come to you with my problems, setbacks, heartaches, or life challenges, you always flip them into something positive. I love that."

My inner self-talk was screaming, *What? Who me? Write a book? I barely can speak proper English with my country self.*

"Oooh, no ma'am, not me, but thanks for the compliment."

Yes, that negative self-talk was straight out of this author's mouth. Nevertheless, my response actually perfectly qualified me to write this book. Why? Because I acknowledged my negative self-talk. Acknowledgement is the number one key to starting your personal journey against your destructive thoughts.

According to the National Science Foundation, the average person has 12,000 to 60,000 thoughts per day. Of those, 95 percent are the same repetitive thoughts we had the day before, and of those thoughts, 80 percent are negative. These negative thoughts have a tremendous impact on our happiness and confidence.

I strongly believe that the negative conversation we have with ourselves is the number one challenge we face daily. This dialogue conquer our desires and causes us to lose our ability to feel complete. We cannot overcome defeat by negative self-talk.

1

Sadly, throughout my life, the majority of my accomplishments were due to my inner pain and negative self-talk. I was constantly fighting to change my thoughts as well as my outcome. Some would say that I was motivated by pain, but it was a way to forget and cover up the discomfort, and to prove my worth to myself and others. I have always worked hard to be the opposite of what my own mother labeled me, what the data about a low-income neighborhood predicted, and what statistics identified as a little black girl in the 'hood who would become a welfare mom.

As I got older, I struggled with the insight and awareness of prejudice against different races. Can you imagine the challenge of not being dark enough for black people and not being light enough for white people? As I became an adult, every failed relationship equaled another "FAILURE" certificate under my belt.

There have been numerous speedbumps, sharp curves, stop signs, caution lights, and road rage on my journey to overcoming negative self-talk. Connecting with my own personal coaches and other like-minded women pursuing similar goals made all the difference on my path to changing my thinking and creating positive results. Instead of saying I couldn't do something, I found a way to make it happen. Instead of feeling defeated and not pursuing my dreams, I overcame my negative mindset and obtained an abundance of success along the way. My path now oozes with positivity and happiness.

Negative Self-Talk

Self-talk is internal dialogue that we have with ourselves. We all engage in self-talk, but the key to success is making sure our self-talk isn't negative. Negative self-talk is directing your thoughts in ways that are unproductive, downbeat, or pessimistic. It impacts your mood, takes away your power, and elevates your anxiety. This "stinkin' thinkin,'" as Zig Ziglar calls it, is an ugly mindset that causes what I call your war wounds. They can include:

- ⮕ always having negative thoughts about yourself. (I am so fat!)
- ⮕ not having any positive thoughts about your future. (My family will never be proud of me.)
- ⮕ saying more of what you can't do than what you can do. (I'll never be able to lose this weight.)
- ⮕ quitting before you begin new ventures. (That new dance routine looks like fun, but why try? I have two left feet.)
- ⮕ being afraid that things will not work in your favor. (I already know I will mess up that recipe. I can't even boil water.)
- ⮕ using terms like I can't, I hate, I'm not good enough, I'm not good at, I want to but, What if, It's too late, and I'm too old.

Here are some other examples of an ugly mindset: You are the owner of an "I hate Mondays" T-shirt. Every Monday, you automatically give yourself that special weekly negative self-talk, ensuring a miserable Monday every week. Or you see a coworker, whom you consider a friend, talking to another coworker who you don't like. You convince yourself through negative self-talk that they are talking about you. Or you are excited about a second date scheduled this weekend, but you received a text message that an emergency came up and he has to cancel. You immediately assume that the cancellation was because you aren't good enough.

We try to ease such mental disappointments with unhealthy habits and patterns, such as chewing ice, binge eating, drinking too much, smoking, and using drugs, to numb the pain and persuade ourselves that we are at peace with our unhappy situation.

I have found that we women spend years questioning ourselves, trying to figure out why we feel powerless. What constantly pushes us into a downward spiral? How can we bring the best of ourselves to the forefront and keep ourselves there?

This transformative workbook will help you learn how to FIRE your negative thoughts and set yourself on a path to a more fruitful way of thinking by hiring a more positive YOU. It's about being the boss over your thoughts by implementing the firing-and-hiring process. I offer it to you as a vehicle to open your mind in an explosive and unique way.

Whether you are working a job, launching a new business, considering furthering your education, or are a stay-at-home mom, you must understand that life challenges and obstacles will come, regardless of the journey you take. You must prepare and strengthen your mind, even as you prepare yourself for all possible outcomes, by eliminating negative thinking and self-talk. I want you to be excited for your current circumstances and your journey ahead; cautious, but willing to take the next step, no matter what! By taking action steps to navigate your thoughts, beliefs, patterns, and self-talk, you increase your chances to fulfill your purpose.

By failing to prepare, you are preparing to fail.

—UNKNOWN

I decided to write *Shift Your Confidence!* to show you and other women, whom I call my Queen Sisters, a new way to control your thoughts. The method I developed to control your negative self-talk requires going deep while still having fun by using my favorite phrase, "U R FIRED! I FIRED DAT AZZ!" as if you were terminating an employee who is not a good fit for your business. Using this phrase is memorable, fun to say, and brings awareness to those unwanted thoughts.

I desire to lift women up and erase the negativity from their thoughts that is keeping them from reaching their ultimate goals in life. This is how it works. THE SCENE: You have been invited to perform your very first speech in front of a crowd of entrepreneur women. You are super excited that you were chosen. You have spent weeks preparing, but you don't feel confident and are still stumbling over your words. You start telling yourself that your audience is more successful than you are and that they will laugh you out of the room. The negative thoughts are so strong that you call and cancel the engagement. You tell yourself you were stupid to even think that you could do it. A more serious issue is that this isn't the first time this has happened. Your negative self-talk has blocked your success for a long period of time. The solution is to FIRE DAT AZZ! Call out your negative self-talk. See it for what it is and the defeat it causes in your life. Then hire a new self-talk thought that supports your success.

My technique is about reversing these war wounds. It's about overcoming life challenges, obstacles, unhealthy habits, and triggers by regaining your voice—or maybe creating a voice that you have never had. It will help you to disrupt that generational curse of the mind, that fear, that inner dialog that causes critical damage and becomes an ongoing pattern in every area of your life—and that many of us think is the norm.

Throughout the workbook I will use my personal voice to influence you, encourage you, and impact your current state of mind. I will also share my lightbulb moments (the moments of spontaneous and instantaneous realizations) to spark your inner light and assure you that you aren't alone.

The *Shift Your Confidence!* workbook is divided into fifteen days, each with step-by-step targets. I share tools that I use daily, and you will learn about some amazing apps available that can help you organize your days and destress your mind. My "Mirror Self-Admiration Chat" was designed for you to start having more positive dialogue with yourself and to congratulate yourself each time you have accomplished a new task. Mindful self-talk workouts will help you to be consistent in changing your negative self-talk, and each activity will prepare you for the next level. Every day includes the following:

- ➲ daily lessons and stories
- ➲ daily activities
- ➲ daily tools
- ➲ daily mirror self-admiration chat

These workouts and activities will help support new growth in your mindset. Ask yourself, How am I waking up to myself daily? How am I showing up in my thoughts? How am I preparing myself for my happiness today, or at this exact moment? How am I empowering myself? How am I staying in control of my power, my voice, and my joy? How am I steering my current circumstances on the road to a lifetime of happiness? My strategies and techniques will help you to find positive answers to these questions and more.

Before we get started, I want you to stop stressing and beating yourself up about your personal struggles with your current way of thinking. Yes, negative self-talk is a fight in itself, but it's a fight that you can win! As you work through the book, I want you to remember that you are the boss over your thoughts! You have all the power to control your self-talk and boost your self-confidence. During the next fifteen days you will take a deep dive into cultivating a mindset of positivity and a can-do attitude. It won't always be easy, and it will require dedicated focus and commitment, but believe me, it will be worth it. I'm going to teach you how to FIRE DAT AZZ!

We all have unshakable confidence within us. We were born with it. Remember, you were born to win! Let's get started! It's time to free your mind!

We all have unshakable confidence within us. We were born with it. Remember, you were born to win! Let's get started! It's time to free your mind!

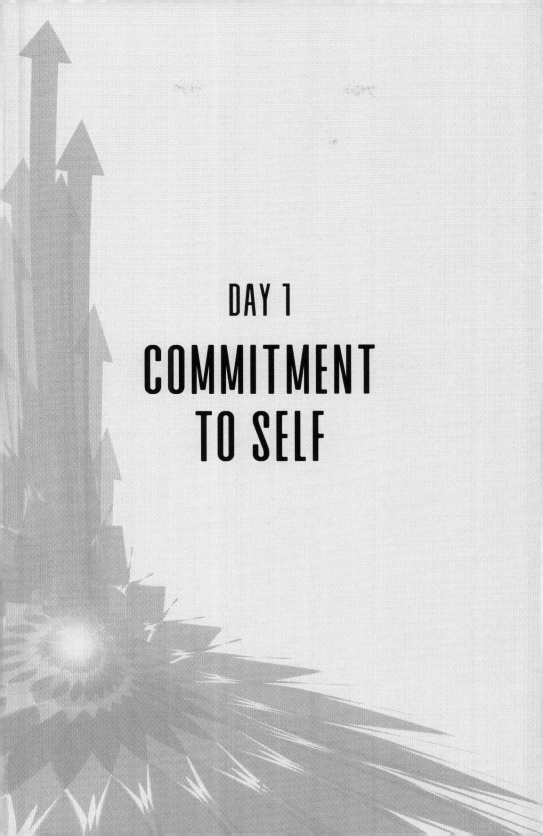

DAY 1

COMMITMENT
TO SELF

DAY 1

COMMITMENT TO SELF

I was the worst when it came to negative self-talk. I constantly brought myself down as I got older. I've always been challenged by committing to my goals, but, I do remember my lightbulb moment as if it were yesterday.

It was the beginning of December, 2009, and I was preparing my New Year's resolution. This year was going to be the best ever. President Obama had just been elected the forty-fourth president of the United States, and I was excited about new beginnings. I had survived my divorce. I talked about a new beginning as a single woman, all the changes I would make, how I was going to stay consistent and achieve all my goals. My thoughts were all positive, and I was on a natural high. Hip hop preacher Eric Thomas says, "Don't talk about it, be about it," and that was my motivation.

I've always loved planning for the new year by doing a vision boards party. The lack of commitment wasn't because of an absence of talent or ability to succeed at a task. It was because of my failure to focus in one area. Success in reaching any goal requires focus.

As I started pursuing my goals, I felt amazing. I was running on pure excitement. My mind and body were ready to get started. But as the months passed, I began to feel overwhelmed. There was never enough time in the day to complete my to-do list. Life challenges constantly came up that I hadn't included in my plan. My expectations were too high to stay focused and succeed at every one of my goals. Then the excuses started negatively attacking my self-talk.

We all want to be our best at whatever we set out to do, but how can you give your all if you are focused on too many tasks? For example, let's say that these are my goals and dreams on my vision board:

- ➲ exercise for thirty minutes four times a week
- ➲ create a better eating habit
- ➲ start new investments
- ➲ start a new business
- ➲ go back to school
- ➲ get rid of my shopping habit
- ➲ learn to ballroom dance

Even though each of these are great goals and can be accomplished, trying to do them all becomes overwhelming. You might become uninterested in them, one at a time, which causes failure and disappointment.

Negative self-talk can start to creep in and give you loads of excuses for not making your goals:

- ➲ My body is too sore to exercise so long and so often.
- ➲ I'm on the road too much to cook, and it's too expensive to eat healthy.
- ➲ I might lose money if I invest.
- ➲ Start-up businesses only have a 10 percent success rate.

- ⮑ I haven't found success with the degrees that I already have, so why go back to school?
- ⮑ I deserve to spend some money on myself.
- ⮑ I'm too old to learn to ballroom dance.

Before you know it, none of the goals are reached, no commitments are made.

After I had failed to reach any of my goals, I had my big lightbulb moment. I started to think about other successful entrepreneurs and celebrities. How do they succeed? What do they focus on? My research showed that:

> Serena Williams focuses on what it takes to be the best tennis player.

> Oprah Winfrey focuses on having a top media empire.

> Beyonce Knowles focuses on being the top artist in the entertainment business.

> Debbi Fields focuses on being the top bakery in the country.

These successful women's focus isn't all over the place. Their focus is totally on their passion and purpose in life. Even though you may have many dream items on your vision board, your focus should be on your purpose and passion. Committing, focusing, and achieving success in your top goals will assist in your reaching the other desires on your vision list.

Using myself as an example, my focus for 2021 goals is to 1) teach women to FIRE their negative self-talk, and 2) write a best-selling book.

Don't pretend that the excuses won't try to attack your thoughts. Remember, negative self-talk is a known fact. My negative thoughts might look like this: 1) they won't listen to me because there are more qualified coaches out there, and 2) I'm not smart or intelligent enough to write a book.

Making a commitment to yourself is the first step. You must also commit to controlling your stinkin' thinkin'!

My new self-talk looks like this: Samantha, today I commit to sharing my experiences to help me teach women to FIRE their negative self-talk. I will achieve this by writing a how-to best-selling book.

Day 1 is about making a commitment to never lose yourself, to avoid overwhelming yourself or setting unachievable high expectations. Make today the last day to come up with excuses to not commit to yourself.

In order to have the best success with any journey, you must start with your own personal commitment. Today's Commitment to Self is designed to set you on a path to positive thinking.

Commitment leads to action. Action brings your dreams closer.

—MARCIA WIEDER

Today's Tool

Today's tool is a template for a commitment letter to yourself so you can create a printable version, and prepare yourself for the journey by being the boss over your thoughts.

Use this template to write a commitment letter to yourself, or create your own.

My Commitment Letter

I, _____ am committed to taking action to strengthen and build my inner thoughts in a positive manner.

I will prioritize my schedule and make time to commit to my fifteen-day guide to the ultimate self-talk workout.

I commit to consistently measuring my progress and growth without having over-the-top expectations.

I will not allow myself to get stuck or be in denial because of my fears, anxieties, or uneasy feelings.

I am ready for the most important battle of my life: eliminating my negative self-talk. I am aware that life challenges will come up, and I commit to being an active participant throughout my journey.

I commit to removing the words *I can't, I hate, I'm not good enough, I'm not good at, it's too late, but what if, I want to but*, and *I'm too old* from my self-talk.

Repeat after me: I am committed! I am a winner! I am strong!

Signed _____

Date _____

Day 1 Workout: Commitment to Self

Now that you have written your commitment letter, take the following steps to make it real.

Step 1: Print, sign, and frame your Commitment to Self. Hang it where you can see it daily as a reminder of your commitment to yourself.

Step 2: Record yourself on your electronic device reading your commitment with confidence. This way you can listen to or watch it at any time you feel your negative self-talk sneaking in your thoughts.

Mirror Self-Admiration Chat

Today, give yourself some self-admiration by saying out loud into the mirror:

I, _____ am so proud of myself for making a commitment to my personal dialogue with myself journey.

Day 1: What an amazing accomplishment! Have a blessed and prosperous day on purpose!

DAY 2

ACKNOWLEDGE YOUR NEGATIVE SELF-TALK

ACKNOWLEDGE YOUR NEGATIVE SELF-TALK

A client who participated in my Intensive 6-Week Confident Shift group program struggled with being aware of her negative self-talk. Her daily workout assignments were usually incomplete because she stated that she was a positive person and didn't have many bad thoughts, especially about herself. The only reason she was there was because her job required proof of her participation in a mindset development class before promoting her to a new position.

During every session, she consistently denied that she engaged in negative self-talk. She would say, "I know that I am enough. I know my worth!" However, it was important that she acknowledge her personal thoughts without needing me or anyone in the class to point them out. Most people go into defense mode if someone points out what they consider their weaknesses. Acknowledgment is an important step toward healing, and this group's focus was healing and mindset growth.

The other participants were open about their negative self-talk, how it originated, and how it held them back. Once this woman acknowledged the challenge she was having in being aware of her negative self-talk, she agreed to participate in a one-on-one session. This allowed us to dive deeper, and it brought out her fear of being too vulnerable. She worked in sales and had to be confident at all times. As we worked privately, I realized that she believed that admitting to the negative self-talk would be a sign of weakness in front of the other participants. She was approaching her journey of self-discovery as a challenge rather than a place to heal.

Once she realized that she was in a safe space to open up and that she was not alone, the wall came down. She finally grasped the fact that she wasn't losing her power by admitting to being aware of her negative self-talk, but rather that she was actually gaining a greater control over the success that she was seeking. Because of her growth, she is now in her dream position at her job and getting great reviews from her clients.

Being stuck or in denial blocks the path to growth and happiness. Sometimes, what stops us is the fear of change, fear of being less-than, or believing that admitting our self-talk is a sign of weakness. Some of us have denied our self-talk for so long that we don't even recognize it or know it's harmful.

Accepting your negative thoughts can be a challenge, but acknowledging this self-talk is the number one key to your mindset growth. It is the beginning process toward self-care of the mind. One of the biggest steps toward healing is knowing how powerful acknowledgment is.

Let's evaluate why you might be afraid to admit your negative self-talk: You fear what other people will think of you. You think that you are the only one with these thoughts. You fear losing your relationship with the person you share your thoughts with, leaving you feeling abandoned or paralyzed. You think that you are not good enough anyway, so why try to improve? These are just possibilities. Your reality may differ.

Solution: FIRE DAT AZZ!

Remember, this is your journey and no one else's. Worrying about other people's opinions of you will block your growth. This journey is all about you. This is your safe space to heal. Moving past your fears is a must. Knowing that you are worthy and that we all have negative thoughts makes this process easier. We are here to learn how to control them together.

This technique consists of catching yourself in the middle of your thoughts and taking back control of your mind. Once you catch your negative thought, them repeat after me: "U R FIRED! I FIRED DAT AZZ!"

This might feel weird in the beginning. If so, you can whisper it. But if you enjoy expressing yourself, then say it out loud: "U R FIRED! I FIRED DAT AZZ!"

Remember You are the boss over your thoughts!

Practice makes progress.

Today's Tool

Keep a pocket journal in your purse, and write down your negative self-talk every time you catch yourself. The Notes app on your phone is a great alternative. This tool is an important beginning of your process. You can also purchase my personal *Confidence Shift* pocket journal on my website.

Day 2 Workout: Take Action

Practice catching yourself saying negative self-talk, and then write it down. Read your negative thought, then write these words in big letters: U R FIRED! I FIRED DAT AZZ! This is a powerful exercise to incorporate daily. (We will go deep into the meaning of these words in the upcoming days.)

Here are some examples:

I can't do anything right. U R FIRED! I FIRED DAT AZZ!

I am not pretty enough. U R FIRED! I FIRED DAT AZZ!

I will stay at home because I am too fat. U R FIRED! I FIRED DAT AZZ!

In the space below, list your negative self-talk as you catch it. After you read through it, repeat to yourself, U R FIRED! I FIRED DAT AZZ!

Mirror Self-Admiration Chat

Today, give yourself some self-admiration by saying out loud into the mirror:

I, _____ am so proud of myself for having the courage to acknowledge my negative self-talk.

Day 2: What an amazing accomplishment. Have a blessed and prosperous day on purpose!

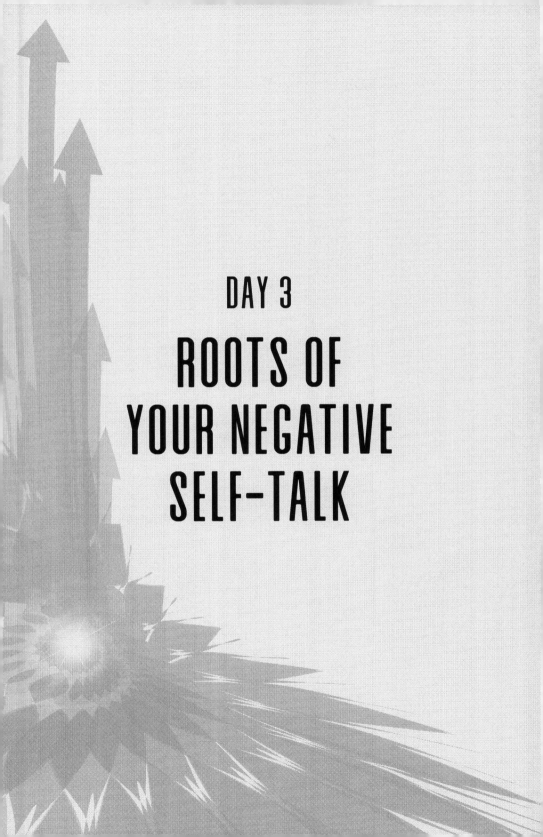

DAY 3

ROOTS OF YOUR NEGATIVE SELF-TALK

DAY 3

ROOTS OF YOUR NEGATIVE SELF-TALK

I grew up in a poor and toxic environment. My stepfather was very abusive toward my mother. His drinking habits got out of hand, and he cheated on my mother constantly. My parents consistently used profanity in the house. Having a voice was unheard of for the children, and the words "I love you" were needed but never used.

As a child, I dreamed of having a large, beautiful mansion with the white-picket-fence type of lifestyle as seen on TV. I just knew that I would grow up to be a famous and wealthy woman one day. I didn't know what I wanted to be because it was embedded in me that my dream was too big and wasn't possible, anyway. And only people with money were famous. I worked hard to succeed in everything, just in case.

I was a very positive child at one time, but I felt like every time I dreamed of something amazing happening in my life, only bad things occurred. My negative thoughts started out with small, simple things. For example, if I was feeling nervous about an exam, I would tell myself, "Samantha, you know you gonna flunk this test." This way, if I *didn't* get an F, then I did pretty well. I thought I had created a new way to feel happy all the time; I was unknowingly using reverse psychology on myself.

My childhood technique was eventually tested by bigger issues that no longer had happy endings, but I still faked it. For example, my dad was an alcoholic. He would be gone the entire weekend then come home, broke and drunk. Unfortunately for the children in the house, my mom would be upset the entire time he was gone. She would punish me for any small thing. But when I prepared myself for the worst, better things seemed to happen. While I lay in my bed in tears each night, instead of praying, I gave myself serious negative self-talks so that the next day would appear better. That was the beginning of my negative self-talk.

To this day, I sometimes struggle with bad thoughts of danger, death, bad accidents, rape, murder, hurt, and harm. This is how I know the extent and impact of negative self-talk. I knew that it was my purpose from God to share this technique with my Queen Sisters around the world.

Most of our negative thoughts stem from our childhood experiences and spiral into our adult life. Psychologist Jean Piaget's theory of cognitive development states that there are four stages of childhood: birth to twenty-four months, two to seven years, seven to eleven years, and adolescence to adulthood. Within these four stages of cognitive development, Piaget points out that the way we think affects all stages of our lives. Many of us have experienced verbal abuse that could be the cause of our negative thinking.

I want to reiterate the importance of knowing that negative thoughts are normal and that you are the boss over your thoughts. You need to be aware of your origin story so that you don't fall into the same old trap over and over again.

Whether your negative self-talk began during those first few critical years of your life or more recently, you allowed someone or something to impact your cognitive thinking. You have adapted to your negative thinking process, and it is affecting your ability to be great. It also affects other aspects of yourself, such as your ability to:

- be a problem solver
- feel good about yourself
- think positive
- know that great things are in store for you
- find joy and happiness in your life

Solution: FIRE DAT AZZ!

Your thoughts control your emotions. When you think negatively, your emotions can cause sadness, depression, anxiety, and worry. When you think positive, your emotions are joyful, happy, excited, and great. This is why I want you to say, U R FIRED! I FIRED DAT AZZ! when you recognize a negative thought. It is humorous and positive at the same time.

> Whatever you hold in your mind on a consistent basis is exactly what you will experience in your life.
>
> —TONY ROBBINS

Today's Tool

Look back over what you've written so far in your pocket journal. Did you see anything different about your self-talk? Keep making notes in your pocket journal every time you catch yourself engaged in negative self-talk. Consistent practice will become a healthy habit.

Day 3 Workout: Identify the Source of Your Negative Self-Talk

Where does your negative self-talk stem from? The purpose of this exercise is to bring more awareness to how your negative self-talk began. In the space below, write a story about a moment in your childhood or in your life that triggered your negative self-talk.

Once you have learned where your negative self-talk originated, you can FIRE DAT AZZ! U R FIRED! I FIRED DAT AZZ!

Mirror Self-Admiration Chat

Today, give yourself some self-admiration by saying out loud into the mirror:

I, _____ am so proud of myself for acknowledging where my negative self-talk stems from.

Day 3: What an amazing accomplishment. Have a Blessed & Prosperous Day on Purpose!

DAY 4

ACKNOWLEDGE YOUR SELF-SABOTAGE

DAY 4

ACKNOWLEDGE YOUR SELF-SABOTAGE

My client Annie is a highly successful entrepreneur who loves what she does. She comes from an exceptionally large family, whom she loves dearly. She is enjoying life and living on top of the world, but it has not always been that way.

Annie once battled with juggling her life as a single mom, full-time student, and a full-time employee. By the time she got home from a long day's work, she didn't have any energy left. She couldn't figure out how to balance the kids' activities, cooking dinner, exercising, studying, and making time for her family and friends. On the weekends, she felt like she had even more to do.

Then her mother became sick, and everyone had to pitch in. She was already overwhelmed and frustrated. With this additional challenge, her grades began to decline, she was never on time for work, she didn't have any time for self-care, and eating out was financially draining her. Her negative self-talk put her in a depressed emotional state. She constantly told herself that time wasn't on her side, that she had nothing to offer anyone, she wasn't smart enough to finish school, and she deserved what she got. Then fear would set in and she would yell, "I give up! I can't do this anymore!" Annie was exhausted.

If she didn't find a healthy balance, everything would fall apart. Coming home to a glass of wine and doing absolutely nothing wasn't working.

Applying multiple coaching techniques helped to break down and organize Annie's daily schedule. She also learned a few things about herself that she hadn't realized: she procrastinated; was paralyzed by stress, leading her to do nothing; and self-sabotaged by her use of negative self-talk. She also discovered that there were plenty of times she could focus on her daily responsibility, but she had used that time to binge-watch her TV shows, scroll through social media, and drink her favorite wine.

Annie didn't have a process. While it was easy for her to follow her work schedule, she didn't create a schedule for herself to balance her studies and her home life. She was engaging in self-sabotage by passively taking steps that prevented her from reaching her goals.

After acknowledging these things, Annie is now back on track. She successfully graduated with honors and started her own business.

What Is Self-Sabotage?

According to Healthline.com, self-sabotage refers to behaviors or thought patterns that hold you back and prevent you from doing what you want to do. In my opinion as a certified life coach, negative self-talk and self-sabotage go hand and hand. Negative self-talk operates in ways that push you to that self-sabotage stage. These acts are unhealthy yet common. It's important to be aware of when you participate in such an act, because there is a great possibility that it is affecting your happiness.

The following behaviors are examples of ways you may engage in self-sabotage:

Replaying events in your head of what you shouldn't have done. For example, you created the perfect healthy diet plan and were sticking to it until you attended a birthday party and couldn't resist trying the punch bowl cake. You became disappointed in yourself, and now you can't stop thinking about it.

Being extremely hard on yourself by putting yourself down, insulting yourself, and repeating harsh, negative self-talk as a result of setting unrealistic goals for yourself. For example, you think, I look fat and slouchy in this family picture because I didn't work out hard enough these last two weeks; or, *I could have done a better job on that work project if I had worked an extra hour every day. I will never be good enough.*

Setting a goal but never getting started, or procrastinating to complete a task. For example, you pick up an application to go to nursing school but never fill it out; or, you have an important deadline but procrastinate by starting the dishwasher, putting on a load of clothes in, or sweeping the floor.

Having plans but letting anxiety set you back. For example, you have been excited all week about a date with a guy that you really like, but you missed getting your hair done, so you decide to cancel and stay home to watch TV alone.

Being uncomfortable with sharing your feelings or fixing your relationship problems. For example, your marriage is on the rocks because instead of talking about an intimacy challenge, you change the subject or avoid the conversation altogether.

Self-sabotage is mostly unintentional and is considered a defense mechanism, meaning that you are safeguarding yourself from hurt and disappointment. However, self-sabotage can affect your career, relationship, health, and finances. The good news is that these behaviors can be controlled. As you learned on Day 2, acknowledgment is key, and that is your focus for now. It's up to you to put your life in order by acknowledging how you get in your own way.

Whether you think you can or t hink you can't, you're right.

Thinking you can't do something or don't have enough time equals automatic procrastination, so there's a slim chance you will get any task done.

As you work through the process of becoming aware of your mindset, your goal is to first acknowledge the problem and then confirm that you aren't passively or actively engaging in self-sabotage.

Solution: FIRE DAT AZZ!

Instead of coming up with reasons why you can't do something or won't even try, we will continue equipping your mind for growth by acknowledging the negative self-talk and asking yourself, "Why?" Why do you feel you are unable to succeed? Is it because you are not sure where to start? Asking the right questions will assist you in finding a solution to your engaging in self-sabotage. We will go deeper into those questions further along in the journey, but for today, just acknowledge when you sabotage yourself and then practice using your new technique and FIRE DAT AZZ!

Don't stand in your own way.

Today's Tool

Try the self-care app called Sparkle, or create a self-care day where you initiate lots of self-love at least once a week for your mind, body, or hobby. For example, write a love letter to yourself, show gratitude in your journal (using affirmation), take a long relaxing bath, do a selfie photo shoot, listen to soft music, put on your favorite lipstick and heels just because, or read a good book.

Treat yourself like your bestie, your ride-or-die partner!

Day 4 Workout: Acknowledge Your Self-Sabotage

List all of the ways that you may unintentionally self-sabotage your goals and dreams, then FIRE DAT AZZ. U R FIRED! I FIRED DAT AZZ!

Here are some examples:

I'm not going to try that, because I might fail. U R FIRED! I FIRED DAT AZZ!

I'm just going to stay in bed instead of running in the marathon that I have been training for weeks for. U R FIRED! I FIRED DAT AZZ! *I am terrible at budgeting, so trying to aim for wealth is useless.* U R FIRED! I FIRED DAT AZZ!

In the space below, list all the ways you self-sabotage. After you read through it, repeat to yourself, U R FIRED! I FIRED DAT AZZ!

Mirror Self-Admiration Chat

Today, give yourself some self-admiration by saying out loud into the mirror:

I, _____, am so proud of myself for not self-sabotaging my goals and dreams.

Day 4: What an amazing accomplishment. Have a blessed and prosperous day on purpose!

DAY 5

RETRAINING
THE MIND

DAY 5

RETRAINING THE MIND

Writing this, my first book, was a huge challenge for me. Even though I had been coaching for years, which doesn't require a certification, I decided to enroll to become a certified life coach at the age of fifty-four. I also took other classes because I desired to have personal testimony for my Queen Sisters. This would be my proof that we are never too old to reach our life goals. During my Speak and Inspire training with Lisa Nicols, she reiterated the importance of creating dialogue. It was like getting approval that I knew what I was talking about.

However, when it came to writing my book, I ran into an unexpected problem. I was trained to ask a lot of yes-or-no questions when I talk one-on-one or to groups of people, so I proceeded to write my book using those techniques. I had written the entire book and proofread it multiple times. It took months. I was super excited and ready to take the next step.

A dear friend recommended an editor who turned out to be an amazing queen. I sent her a copy of my book, and we scheduled our first Zoom meeting. I was so excited. She praised me on my writing, and I was smiling from ear to ear. She continued with more compliments on what I had written. However, before I could take another breath, that big cutthroat word came from her lips: "*But!*" OMG, no she didn't!

She pleasantly explained to me the difference between presenting a speech and writing a book. The use of dialogue is great for writing speeches, but it doesn't work for a book. She explained that monologue teaching, where there is only output because the reader can't actually answer to me, is used for writing the type of book that I was aiming for. Then she said, "We still have a lot of work to do!" She instructed me to change this, elaborate here, be consistent here, delete that, rephrase this, rewrite this, move that . . . and the list went on.

You can imagine the negative self-talk that rose up in my mind. I had to completely retrain my thinking while writing this book. For the next three weeks, I used my own technique on myself over a hundred times.

You are the BOSS over your thoughts!
U R FIRED! I FIRED DAT AZZ!

Today's focus is to nourish your mind with positive thoughts by retraining your way of thinking. Retraining your mind is a challenge in itself, but I have some amazing tips for you in the upcoming days. Yes, it is a process, but I know you can do it! We will do it together.

For every negative thought you have, try to change it to something positive. For example, if you say, "I don't have time to go back to school," try saying, "Let's see how I can make this work in the time I do have." Or, instead of saying, "I am not a good writer," try saying, "The more I practice writing, the more I will improve." Retraining your mind is all about changing your perspective. Once you change your perspective, you'll realize that there are things you once struggled with that you can now do with ease.

In one of my self-talk coaching sessions, I talked about how "the mind is a terrible thing to waste," which is a famous quote by the United Negro College Fund. We talked about the importance of memory and how, whether long or short term, our beautiful brains are one of the things we can control. In fact, you can influence your brain to do anything you want it to do. You can influence it to be as powerful as you want it to be, and as successful as you wish. You can control your stinkin' thinkin'!

You are in charge of that negative self-talk that goes on in your mind. You must learn how to control it. Now that you have acknowledged your negative self-talk, can recognize it when it occurs, and know where it came from, it's time to fix the issue by retraining your mind. In today's workout, you will continue to practice changing your negative self-talk to positive self-talk.

Talk to yourself like you would to someone you love.

—BRENÉ BROWN

Today's Tool

One of my favorite free affirmation app tools is called Daily Affirmation. I recommend that you download it and give it a try. Also, write your favorite affirmation on all of your mirrors using dry erase marker so you will see it daily.

Day 5 Workout: Fire That Negative Self-Talk

You have been practicing firing negative self-talk for the last three days. Today, you will practice reversing your thinking from negative to positive. Whenever you FIRE those "employees" because they are not a great fit, you have to hire new ones. I call this "The Firing/ Hiring Process."

Here are some examples of negative self-talk that you saw in Day 2, along with a positive statement to replace each one:

I can't do anything right. U R FIRED! I FIRED DAT AZZ! Replace that thought with, "I can do anything I put my mind to."

I am not pretty enough. U R FIRED! I FIRED DAT AZZ! Replace that thought with, "I am beautiful from head to toe."

I will stay at home because I am too fat. U R FIRED! I FIRED DAT AZZ! Replace that thought with, "I have amazing curves."

In the space below, make a list of your negative self-talk. Then FIRE them and hire positive thoughts. After you read through it, repeat to yourself, U R FIRED! I FIRED DAT AZZ! Incorporate this exercise daily.

Mirror Self-Admiration Chat

Today, give yourself some self-admiration by saying out loud into the mirror:

I, _____, am so proud of myself for learning to reverse my negative thoughts.

Day 5: What an amazing accomplishment. Have a blessed and prosperous day on purpose!

DAY 6

SELF-REFLECTION
#1

DAY 6

SELF-REFLECTION #1

Today is a day to self-reflection, focusing on your journey thus far. Reflect on your progress in your awareness of negative thoughts and self-talk. This week's focus has been on acknowledgment of your negative thoughts and how to shift them to positive.

Things to remember:

- ➲ Your commitment to yourself must come first.
- ➲ Your mind controls your entire life.
- ➲ You are the BOSS over your thoughts.

The goal today is to recognize and reflect on your biggest inner shift. We will dive deeper in the days to come.

Reflection is looking back so that the view looking forward is even clearer.

Today's Tool

Use the questionnaire in today's workout to rate your acknowledgment development stage.

Day 6 Workout: Self-Reflection #1

Today is the time to reflect on how you have progressed in acknowledging your negative self-talk.

Questionnaire

Rate your progress after participating in days 1 through 5 using the scale below. Make a note of the points you give each question, then add them up at the end.

Never (0 pts) Sometimes (1 pt) Above average (2 pts) Most of the time (3 pts) All of the time (5 pts)

> 1) I am fully committed to my journey of transforming my negative self-talk.
>
> 2) I have acknowledged and evaluated my self-talk daily.
>
> 3) I have consistently fired my negative self-talk with the phrases, U R FIRED! I FIRED DAT AZZ!
>
> 4) I can pinpoint areas of my life in the past where some of my negative thoughts stem from.
>
> 5) I am able to recognize when I am self-sabotaging.
>
> 6) Retraining my mind is working for me.
>
> 7) I am excited to learn more.

TOTAL: _____

0 pts = no progress

1 to 7 pts = very little progress

8 to 14 pts = some progress (I recommend you re-read days 1 through 5)

15 to 21 pts = moving in the right direction

22 to 28 pts = amazing job

29 to 35 pts = You are 100 percent ready for the next step in your journey.

Day 6 Bonus Workout

Today you get a bonus workout! In the space provided, write some notes and thoughts that support your self-reflection and self-love.

Notes to Self:

Mirror Self-Admiration Chat

Today, give yourself some self-admiration by saying out loud into the mirror:

I, _____, am so proud of myself for beginning my inner shift.

Day 6: What an amazing accomplishment. Have a blessed and prosperous day on purpose!

DAY 7

DIGGING DEEPER– THE ROOTS OF YOUR NEGATIVE SELF-TALK

DAY 7

DIGGING DEEPER – THE ROOTS OF YOUR NEGATIVE SELF-TALK

I have a very close friend named Melissa who, from the outside, seems like she has it all together. She has an amazing family and successful career, but what didn't show was that she was struggling in her marriage. She believed that a marriage should be a partnership but couldn't engage in a true relationship with her husband. She struggled with control issues that were hurting their commitment to one another. As I was writing this book and talking through some of my workout ideas, she shared her story with me. After a lot of self-reflection and some serious work on her self-awareness, Melissa told me that she realized that the root of the problem stemmed from her parents.

This was shocking to me because I had met her parents. They had been together for years and were very loving and incredibly supportive. They desired for Melissa to find her path and live a healthy and prosperous life. But the problem was the dynamic of her parents' relationship—her father was the provider and her mother was the caregiver—yet this was a negative memory for her.

Her dad showed his love by giving. He bought every nice house that they had. Every new house was bigger and better than the previous home. He bought her mom a new car every couple of years, handled things financially, and was supportive of Melissa's education. He was also in attendance for all of the major events in her life. However, all Melissa saw was a woman who was totally dependent on a man and did as she was told, a woman who either had no say or acquiesced in which house they bought or which car was picked out for her.

The negative self-talk Melissa played out in her head included, "I'm never depending on a man," "No man is ever going to control me," and "Men can't be trusted to run everything." She didn't realize how this self-talk affected her until she was married. She had a need to control everything. Arguments went on for days, until her husband gave in to her way of how raise their children, her financial decisions for the home they bought, and her choice of vehicles they purchased. She had turned into her father. Eventually, her husband had had enough and threatened to leave. Thank God, she realized what she was doing before it was too late.

Identifying her origin story helped Melissa to understand why she couldn't truly partner with her husband, which then helped her to look at ways to change the negative self-talk and connect with her husband on a different level.

Psychologists agree that negative events have a greater impact on the brain than positive ones, so it makes sense that the negativity we experience in our lives stays with us and can have a powerful effect. You may not be aware of it, but you are replaying those negative experiences over and over again. You know how kids can remember every negative thing their moms ever said to them but struggle to recall all the praise and support they give them? Unfortunately, this is normal because that is how our brains work.

As you will recall, I didn't feel connected as a child. I didn't feel loved or protected because of my home life. Those feelings caused me to believe that I wasn't worthy of love or protection, which led me to make bad choices in my adult relationships. What's even worse is that sometimes I believed that I was getting what I deserved. My childhood experiences caused and contributed to my stinkin' thinkin'. As I got older, I continued to search for my worth, but I failed to focus on me and instead focused on how I *thought* I should act and what the world said I should be. I failed to look at the root cause of my thoughts and how they were causing my ugly mindset.

Today, you will be diving deeper into your origin story, the roots of your negative self-talk, to help you understand why you think the way you do. This will help you to retrain your mind to stop the negative self-talk. Knowing your origin story is important because it contributes to your negative self-talk. Our negative experiences stick with us and have an influence on our behavior, decisions, and relationships.

Just like we have to acknowledge our negative self-talk, we must also acknowledge the factors that contributed to or caused it. I won't lie to you and tell you this will be an easy task. You might have to remember experiences that were painful for you. You might have to own up to missteps in your past. But this is necessary because, just like you have to acknowledge that you have negative thoughts, you also have to acknowledge WHY you have negative thoughts so your past can no longer have control over your present or future.

A people without the knowledge of their past history, origin and culture is like a tree without roots.

—MARCUS GARVEY

Today's Tool

Cleanse your body daily by tracking your water intake with an app called Drink Water Reminder and Diet. As you drink water, take this time to acknowledge those negative thoughts. It's time to figure out if you have truly moved on from the pain of past experiences. Letting go of past pain, fear, and anger can be hard, but you owe it to yourself. It is an empowering step that will help you focus more on the present and refocus your mindset from negativity to present and future positivity.

Day 7 Workout: Your Origin Story

We all have several areas in our past that led us to develop our negative self-talk, but sometimes one time period or event really stands out. The purpose of this workout is for you to take a deep dive into one of the areas or events in your past that led you to have negative self-talk. Write down your memorable personal origin story in the space provided.

Your Story:

Mirror Self-Admiration Chat

Today, give yourself some self-admiration by saying out loud into the mirror:

I, _____, am so proud of myself for being able to dive deep into the origin of my pain in order to learn where my negative self-talk came from.

Day 7: What an amazing accomplishment. Have a blessed and prosperous day on purpose!

DAY 8

DIGGING DEEPER–
THE COURAGE
TO CHANGE

DAY 8

DIGGING DEEPER – THE COURAGE TO CHANGE

Sharniece's mother and father divorced when she was only four years old. Her mother was a hair stylist and her father was a drug dealer. Nevertheless, Sharniece was a daddy's girl. Even though her father promised to never have Sharniece around his illegal business affairs, she was educated on the entire process. As she got older, she was exposed more and more to the lifestyle of easy money. Men within her father's circle were attracted to Sharniece and pursued relationships with her. She loved the attention. They respected her because of who her father was. In her mind, drug dealers were the only type of men who amounted to what her dad was, and she was only good enough for a man who had the same qualities as her dad. A man who could wine and dine her, protect her, and love their future child, and who reminded her of her dad, became her type.

Sharniece eventually went off to college out of state. She was a very smart young lady, and majored in finance. Her campus tour guide, John, showed interest in her from the first moment they met, but he was not her type. John was of average height, a bookworm, and a true gentleman. She looked at him as a friend.

One weekend, Sharniece met Darnell, the man whom she thought was her dream guy at a sorority party. He was funny, athletic, popular, tall, and handsome. He was also the campus drug dealer. Of course, all of this added up to make Darnell a perfect semblance of her father. The relationship ended a few months later because Darnell decided to change his life to protect his future career.

Sharniece moved on and started dating Big Money, a dealer who didn't attend the college. Even though he became emotionally abusive, Sharniece stayed in the relationship throughout the next year. She thought this was what she needed to feel complete. Big Money had women everywhere and pretended they were customers. His father was a big dealer as well, and taught his son how to use a tactic called blame shifting to manipulate Sharniece and keep her in control.

As the abuse Sharniece suffered got worse, so did her dialogue with herself. Sharniece was now broken. She felt tiny, weak, worthless, and thought everything was her fault. She decided to talk to her roommate about her situation, and her roommate invited Sharniece to my private Facebook group. She listened in on our Wednesday night live call, when the topic was "Attracting the Wrong Guy." She was struggling to find the courage to change her mindset and know her worth.

Later, Sharniece told me that the message that gave her the courage to change was, "We don't attract the wrong guy; we accept the wrong guy because we don't know our worth, even after seeing the red flags."

The Courage to Change Your Relationship

As women, we have to realize that we are the boss over our thoughts and are in control of our happiness. We have the pleasure of choosing to go or not go on that second, third, and fourth date. Pay attention, and recognize the patterns you have that aren't beneficial to your happiness. It's important to have the courage to speak up and have your voice, especially when you see the red flags. Acknowledge if your "type" is equal to your worth. Your happiness matters. Change means being happier than you are right now.

Today's story mentioned blame shifting. Blame shifting is when someone shifts the blame from themselves to others. It is largely used as a control mechanism. I'm sure you know the term "nagging." It is used against another to dismiss their voice. For example, your partner might say that you constantly nag him, but what is really happening is that your partner does not want to communicate or make changes in the partnership to bring the two of you happiness. He tells you to stop nagging him, shifting the blame from his inability to communicate well onto you, as if you are the problem. The real problem, though, is that your needs are not being heard or discussed. Having a successful relationship means being able to take the time to learn each other's love language.

The Courage to Change Your Self-Talk

Today's focus is to make change by taking action on an entirely new level to eliminate the self-talk that has been haunting you for the majority of your life. At this point, you have already participated in a few U R FIRED! I FIRED DAT AZZ! workouts by exploring your own negative self-talk difficulties. Take a minute to celebrate yourself, because I know that your journey isn't easy. You should be truly proud of the progress you have made. Stand up and give yourself a big old-fashioned hug! You are amazing!

Now, let's dive even deeper into change. I want to talk about the courage necessary to change your habits without ever thinking about it. You have already had one big opportunity of courage by digging deeper into your origin story yesterday. You looked at the origins of what makes you engage in negative self-talk. I know that it wasn't easy to acknowledge, and it took courage to face some things in your past, but you did it.

Changing your self-talk without thought consists of self-development, which involves changing your environment. Take a serious look around at your circle and acknowledge things that trigger unwanted self-talk and habit. This is where the courage to change comes in. To support this change, post positive affirmations around your home. I personally have "I AM ENOUGH" posted on all of my mirrors. If you desire to lose weight but love junk food, replace the junk foods in your pantry and refrigerator with healthy foods. Changing your environment is a powerful way to eliminate undesirable self-talk.

Changing your self-talk can also consist of having the courage to stand up to loved ones who partake in part of the problem. For example, you talk to your childhood friend Sandra at least once a week. You love Sandra to death, but during your analysis of your origin story you realized that she has contributed to your negative self-talk. You had a lisp growing up that she teased you about constantly. She still makes little shady comments, and has you convinced that you are a terrible public speaker, which is hindering your growth and your ability to change your self-talk. The next time Sandra calls, you have to have the courage to tell her how her comments have affected you. In order to have the courage to change your self-talk, you need the support from your friends and family.

The Courage to Change Alone

You must have the courage to face your journey alone. I recently read 50 Cent's book *Hustle Harder, Hustle Smarter*. I encourage you to pick up a copy. He shares a series of events and actions that helped (and almost hindered) his journey as an entrepreneur. I won't tell you all of the good details of this book, but I will share an important lesson and powerful tip I took from it: During your journey of changing your habits, you cannot be afraid of outgrowing people. While you work on and improve yourself, you will notice that the people around you will still be comfortable with where they are. I want you to recognize that you are in a place in life where people will become envious of your journey, but don't allow that to stop you from making necessary changes. Everyone won't elevate with you. Your journey might consist of only you!

Yes, change is scary! Your self-talk can take your mind two ways: 1) You can be full of excitement and feeling like a winner on top of the world (so rewarding!) or, 2) you can feel like a total failure, like you took an unnecessary risk and now everyone is giving you the "I told you so" look. It's your choice! Change can be an amazing experience if you really want it.

The Courage to Change and Commit

You must have the courage to commit to your goals. You must be ready to walk the walk and talk the talk. Commitment to this journey might mean that you have to make some uncomfortable changes to see change through to the end. Part of commitment is understanding that there may be consequences at the end of this journey that you didn't anticipate. You have already learned that you might lose some relationships along the way, but that might just be the tip of the iceberg. Let me give you an example of how the courage of commitment can come into play.

As we already talked about, sometimes our environment contributes to our negative self-talk. Maybe we have an unsupportive boss.

Maybe we can't get ahead at work and figure it is a self-fulfilling prophecy of thinking we don't deserve a good life. Having the courage to change may mean relocating if it's possible and necessary. Your negative self-talk may say, "I don't want to relocate because it is so far away," or, "I don't want to move away from my friends and family." You can change your self-talk to give you the courage to make the change to move to an environment where positive self-talk is encouraged and supported. Commit to positive change!

The courage of commitment requires you to show up fully and consistently until you reach your goal. Showing up fully means being authentic. As I was growing up, I saw all these women who had a smile on their face no matter what was going on. But the harder I looked, the more I could see that their smiles were fake, just like mine. To change my fake smile into a real one, I had to have the courage to commit to real change. My coach helped me along the way, and I'm here to help you! Working through this book is a first step, but actively engaging in the steps needed to change is the hard part. Your mind will make excuses for why you can't commit, for why you can't make change. But always remind yourself that you are a prize. Commit to yourself and know that you are strong enough to finish this journey.

The Courage to Change Your Fears

Fear handicaps our courage to make changes in our lives for the better. There are many types of fear: fear of rejection, change, insects, height, death, failure, and so on. Having courage doesn't mean that you are fearless. Fear is mostly imagination; we tend to make fear happen. We even manage to create our fears. Having courage means standing up against your fears. Fear for me is like watching television or going to the movies. I don't like scary movies, so I change the channel and watch an action or romance movie. Whenever I go to the movies, I don't choose a scary movie because I'm in control of what I put into my spirit. Refusing to control what goes on in your thoughts can be damaging. Fear is a choice, and we all have it. This is why I am constantly reiterating that you are the boss over your thoughts.

When I lack courage and fear attempts to step back in my life, my personal quote is, "Fear moves you forward while you remove fear," meaning you use fear, you don't let fear use you. Use fear to move you forward in a positive way while also using fear to remove any negative self-talk.

Every day, every minute, you have the power to choose.

—LISA NICHOLS

Today's Tool

Install the Courage and Strength Quotes app on your phone. Strengthen your courage by starting with small things. Having the courage to change simply means taking action. Courage is the ability to not allow your fear to control or paralyze you. Courage can be built with practice. You can practice courage by volunteering. When something comes up at church, work, or with family, have the courage to go first. Here are some examples:

- ➲ Church: Have the courage to be the first to volunteer to pass out fliers in the neighborhood.
- ➲ Work: Have the courage to be the first to volunteer to oversee a small project.

⊃ Family: Have the courage to be the first volunteer for a family reunion event.

Day 8 Workout: Making Positive Changes

Today you are adding courage to your daily routine. List areas where you desire to strengthen your courage. Start with baby steps. Most importantly, have the courage to change your self-talk. Remember to FIRE DAT AZZ! No debating! Release the fear and feel free! Here are some examples to help you FIRE those fears:

I need this promotion, but it requires being on the roof, and I'm afraid of heights. U R FIRED! I FIRED DAT AZZ! Take small steps to face and overcome your fears. Use breathing techniques, practice mindfulness, or see your doctor for anxiety medication.

There is this guy at the gym who I would love to get to know, but I fear getting rejected. U R FIRED! I FIRED DAT AZZ! Remind yourself of your worth; it would be his loss if he wasn't interested.

It's your turn. Write down areas where you want to strengthen your courage:

Mirror Self-Admiration Chat

Today, give yourself some self-admiration by saying out loud into the mirror:

I, _____, am so proud of myself for having the courage to remove the fears that have been holding me back from my destiny.

Day 8: What an amazing accomplishment. Have a blessed and prosperous day on purpose!

DAY 9

DIGGING DEEPER-SABOTAGE THE SELF-SABOTAGE

.

DAY 9

DIGGING DEEPER – SABOTAGE THE SELF-SABOTAGE

Stella is a wife and mother of four very young children, ages three, five, seven, and eight. Thursday is her grocery shopping day because the stores are less crowded, fresh new coupons come out in her area, and her husband is off work and watches the children.

We all know that getting kids to eat healthy foods can feel almost impossible and that sugary foods lead to behavior problems. Being a mother of four, Stella struggles with her weight. When her family eats unhealthy foods, it is a challenge for her to eat healthy foods herself. She had already acknowledged how and why she was sabotaging her weight journey but couldn't figure out how to change it.

We had already been working on her mindset in my private women's Facebook group, but in order to reach her weight goal, she had to stop her self-sabotaging habits. She started by dissecting her current meal plan, making some healthy changes, and aiming for consistency. Together we made a list of healthy foods that her kids and husband liked. We found some new recipes that used those items, and added the items to her grocery list. For example, the kids love fruits, which are healthy sugars. She added organic whole fruits to their breakfast, and removed sugary cereal. She chose healthy foods like bananas, oatmeal with healthy toppings, eggs, and nuts.

Stella said that from the time she stepped into the grocery store, she began repeating powerful quotes that she learned in her sessions and that had embedded in her memory, such as "I am the BOSS over my own thoughts." Every time she looked at unhealthy foods, she said, "U R FIRED! I FIRED DAT AZZ!" She had had a major lightbulb moment and was so excited to tell me that she couldn't wait for our next session. She said, "My confidence has shifted in a major way. Usually, I despise going to the grocery store because it usually takes up two hours of my day. But today was different."

The most amazing thing was, she would always secretly sit in her car after shopping and sabotage her diet by treating herself to her favorite pack of chocolate chip cookies. That day, the thing she was most proud of was that she successfully avoided her usual guilt routine without even thinking about it.

Whenever you start to see a warning sign of self-sabotage, it is time to STOP! BREATHE! REGROUP! *SABOTAGE THE SELF-SABOTAGE!* Have the courage to move on. Fire those negative thoughts that keep you from knowing your worth. See yourself as the strong queen that you are.

Self-sabotage comes in many forms, including avoidance, failing to prioritize, and procrastination. It can even be negative self-talk itself. Webster defines sabotage as an act or process tending to hamper or hurt. When we self-sabotage, we make decisions that prevent us from reaching our goals or truly engaging in the process. Recall the saying, "If at first you don't succeed, try, try again." When we self-sabotage, the saying is more like, "Don't even try to succeed; if you try and fail, you'll find ways not to try again."

Why We Self-Sabotage

To understand why we self-sabotage, it helps to understand what dopamine is and how it participates in self-sabotage. Dopamine is a neurotransmitter, or a chemical messenger, that stimulates the pleasure box in the brain. Without getting technical, it's a feel-good hormone—which is good, until you become addicted to substances or behaviors that trigger it. Dopamine is like a reward system; think about when you reward your loving furry animal with a treat, and he obeys because he wants more.

Dopamine can control you in negative ways, too. Feeling disappointed or sorry for yourself, such as when you tell yourself, "What was I thinking?" or "Why bother; I might as well give up," lowers your dopamine. When this happens, your body seeks for ways to feel better, and you subconsciously comfort yourself with unhealthy behaviors. This can lead to bad habits like excessive drinking or shopping, smoking, comfort eating, and sex with someone you are not interested in or who is not good for you. All of these behaviors come from trying to comfort yourself, but they only make things worst in the long run.

Knowing your triggers is valuable, and will help you to keep off the roller coaster in your mind. You can use this knowledge to sabotage the self-sabotage within you. Dopamine helps regulate your emotions, but you have to remember that you are the boss over your thoughts. If not, you may continue to self-sabotage.

Self-sabotage is a silent killer of your limited belief. In order to stop self-sabotaging, you have to acknowledge and know what you are doing, and why. You have to ask yourself what you want and determine what is preventing you from getting it. If your answer includes actions that are in your control, you have to then ask yourself if you are engaging in behavior that prevents you from getting what you want.

Solution: FIRE DAT AZZ!

The solution is you. You have the information. You have a choice. Whether you choose to grow or stay comfortably where you are by not making any changes in your life, it's okay. There is no wrong answer. This is about what makes you happy and brings you joy. If you choose to grow and soar like an eagle, you risk losing everything: your friends, your family, your job, your sanity. If you choose to stay where you are, just keep doing what you are doing. You can decide to continue living an unfulfilled life, wondering "what if?" Or you can banish those negative thoughts that hold you back: U R FIRED! I FIRED DAT AZZ! It is your choice.

Let's say you struggle with time management. You are planning to start a business, but your weakness is staying on task and remaining focused. How would you tackle this problem? This is when the self-doubt and negative self-talk usually kick in, because your mind doesn't always go into solution mode when things get difficult. You automatically think you don't have enough time. What strategies could you come up with instead of sabotaging your business? You can start by firing that azz, of course: U R FIRED! I FIRED DAT AZZ! I love it! Next, instead of saying "I don't have enough time," say, "How can I effectively use the time I have?" Then figure out why you struggle with time management. Is it the lack of planning or resources? So, then what? You have no choice but to go into solution mode. You must create a working schedule that allows you to keep track of things.

Acknowledging and being aware of your self-sabotage isn't enough, though. You have to constantly reflect on your actions so that you don't fall back into those same patterns. Let's go back to the quote, "If at first you don't succeed, try, try again." Consider the actual words used, "don't succeed," and "try again." In the first part of the quote, you see an example of reflective thinking. The saying acknowledges the possibility of failing—which can be viewed as negative thinking—but then it immediately offers reassurance that even if your efforts don't work the first time, you are willing to continue to try. Just the thought of "I'm willing to try again" or "I will get what I want" can help you to overcome self-sabotage.

Let's talk about the power of affirmations in helping to sabotage self-sabotage. You have to be able to see your success. It has to be reachable in your mind. For example, one of my mentors posted an affirmation on Facebook that said, "You deserve to be a multimillionaire." You have to speak it repeatedly until you succeed in your mind visually. When I speak it, I say, "Samantha Hill deserves to be a multimillionaire," or "Samantha Hill is a multimillionaire."

For my spiritual warriors, affirmations that you can visualize are the key when quoting your favorite scriptures! For example, I quote Psalm 23, and verses 5 and 6 are my favorite. I always add my name and visualize it.

Thou preparest a table before *Samantha Hill* in the presence of mine enemies: thou anointest *Samantha Hill's* head with oil; *Samantha Hill's* cup runneth over. Surely goodness and mercy shall follow *Samantha Hill* all the days of her life, and *Samantha Hill* will dwell in the house of the Lord forever.

Using affirmations with visualization can help you to sabotage the self-sabotage. Implement this practice into your daily routine. Train your brain to succeed daily.

> ## If you can see it and believe it, it is a lot easier to achieve it.
>
> —OPRAH WINFREY

Today's Tool

Be mindful, and focus on negating your self-sabotage by letting go of your limiting belief and replacing it with the belief that you can achieve what you focus on. For example, if you grew up in a poor, single-parent environment and your mother never made over $30,000, your limited belief might be that you will follow in her footsteps and never go beyond that. Change your outcome by believing you can. Continue using your apps for motivation.

Whenever you feel on edge, STOP! BREATHE! REGROUP! *SABOTAGE THE SELF-SABOTAGE!*

Day 9 Workout: Speak It into Existence

For today's workout, you will use take of the negative self-talk expressions you wrote down in previous days and turn them into positive affirmations that you will say to yourself each day to strengthen and retrain your mind. Your affirmations can be visible somewhere in your home. Add them to your calendar on your cell phone to get notifications, and place them on your refrigerator, a desk area where you work, in your car, in your wallet, or right here in this book. Remember to visualize it. What can you see?

Below are some commonly used negative self-talk phrases, followed by positive affirmations. Revise them for your particular situation.

➲ Negative self-talk: I want to, but . . .

- o Positive affirmation: The only "buts" in my life are the ones I create. I know that I can do _____ if I believe in myself and know that I am capable.

- o Positive affirmation: I am living a life of purpose and happiness. I am ready to explore my passions and chase my dreams.

➲ Negative self-talk: What if (bad things) happen?

- o Positive affirmation: I am the architect of my life. I am working on building my foundation by _____, and I will choose the contents of my "house." Negativity has no place here.

- o Positive affirmation: I am not afraid of failure. I learn from my mistakes, and have the power to turn failures into positive results.

➲ Negative self-talk: I can't because . . .

- o Positive affirmation: I can do _____. Even though there may be challenges, I can overcome anything put in my way.

- o Positive affirmation: My ability to conquer any challenge or obstacle is limitless; my potential to succeed is infinite.

➲ Negative self-talk: There is no use trying to . . .

- o Positive affirmation: Nothing is impossible. If I want to do _____, I can and I will.

○   Positive affirmation: I am enough. I am stronger than I look, and I trust my abilities.

➲   Negative self-talk: I will eventually give up, anyway.

○   Positive affirmation: I am responsible for devising my life's master plan. I have prepared this plan to do _____, and I will complete it.

○   Positive affirmation: I know exactly how I'll get this done, and I have a plan for progress. I can and will succeed.

Use these examples to create your own affirmations. Keep them with you daily, as this is one of the best ways to retrain your mind and way of thinking. As you continue to push positive thoughts into your brain, you will notice a change in how your brain will work for you by encouraging those thoughts.

Mirror Self-Admiration Chat

Today, give yourself some self-admiration by saying out loud into the mirror:

I, _____, am so proud of myself for learning to speak encouraging thoughts in my life.

Day 9: What an amazing accomplishment. Have a blessed and prosperous day on purpose!

DAY 10

DIGGING DEEPER– USING WAR WOUNDS TO RETRAIN THE MIND

DAY 10

DIGGING DEEPER – USING WAR WOUNDS TO RETRAIN THE MIND

One cloudy night, while lightning and thunder raged fiercely outside, we turned the television off; my husband and I were both raised to believe that you don't watch TV in that type of weather. As we sat there, I spotted an old scar on his hand and asked him, "What happened?" We began laughing and talking about the scars on our bodies and how we got them throughout our lives. I noticed that he talked about his scars with pride; when I talked about mine, a sadness came over me. Suddenly, I realized that each scar on our bodies told a story. A joyful smile came to my face, and happiness rushed throughout my body. All my negative thoughts from my scars were now reminders of positive experiences that had taught me lessons.

Retraining your mind the right way brings acceptance, happiness, pleasure, and joy into your life. Today I will focus on how we women unconsciously and consciously tend to compare our bodies to other women as a result of our culture, using scars as examples. Society tells us that we should look a certain way. Social media, magazines, and television are some of the media that dictate what is considered the norm. If you are not careful, such messages can rob you of your happiness. Negative self-talk can also destroy confidence.

Today you will work toward retraining your mind to get that confidence back. Bodies come in different sizes, shapes, colors, and scars—and we all are beautifully made. Your body is part of who you are! It represents your struggles as well as your successes. You are a survivor! I call such marks and scars "war wounds" because each of them tells a story.

War Wounds

Whether from childhood clumsiness, accidents, or birth, the war wounds of bruises, marks, scars, broken bones, and birth defects tell your amazing story. I want to tell you some of my stories.

I have had a nickel-size scar on my knee since childhood; it was a half-dollar size when I got it. Every time I fell—usually off my bike—I landed on the same spot on my knee, reopening it. My negative self-talk told me that I was super clumsy. Now that I have retrained my thoughts, I refer to it as my amazing childhood war wound.

Mothers usually have some kind of scar that represents every childbirth, such as dark spots, loose skin, cellulite, masculine chin hairs, and stretch marks. I'm a mother of four, three girls and a boy. All of my girls were gentle on my body, but my son, the youngest, showed no mercy. I have a huge stretch mark in the middle of my stomach underneath my navel, and there is no hiding it. He made sure that he made his mark before coming out. It is definitely a war wound that I am proud to carry.

Many of us carry wise women war wounds, and it is important that we carry these wisdom wounds with pride. At one time I was afraid of getting older, and I sure wasn't in any hurry to get wrinkles. Now I know that my hanging, wrinkled skin represents all the wisdom that God has allowed me to gain and share with the younger generation. There is nothing more unique than a wise woman full of wisdom to share, as they did in the Bible days.

Retraining Your Mind

Now that you understand some of the ways that we women put down our bodies, let's look at how you can retrain your mind to bring more happiness and peace into your life.

Think of retraining your mind as learning to ride a bike. You started with training wheels, and at some point, you took off the training wheels. You got on, pushed your foot forward, and tried to pedal, but each time you would fall off. You kept falling and sometimes felt like you would never learn how to ride. You pushed on, though, and one day you kept pedaling and didn't fall. You did two things to learn to successfully ride that bike: you had determination, and you were consistent. Retraining your mind is no different from learning to ride a bicycle.

There are multiple ways to retrain your mind. One of the best ways is with determination, which is different from commitment. In Day 8 we talked about the courage of commitment. A commitment is pledging to do something; in this case, pledging to yourself to be the best version you can be. Determination is deciding that you will do what it takes to change, which drives you to commit. It also keeps you on course as you walk your path.

Believe that you can and decide that you will. It's all about the way you think. Maybe you look at yourself in the mirror and are shocked because your favorite jeans no longer fit. You think, *I've gained too much weight, I'm no longer attractive.* You have to learn how to balance your expectations and be determined to stay positive regardless of your unintentional negative thoughts. Push upbeat thoughts to the forefront of your mind and say, "My health is more important than anything. I got this, and I can and will lose the weight."

New Year's resolutions are another example of determination. Usually, at the beginning of every year, we focus on a new start. It's like a reset button that we all believe we need. We then determine to reach some set goal. As racing driver Mario Andretti said, "Desire is the key to motivation, but it is determination and commitment to an unrelenting pursuit of your goal—a commitment to excellence—that will enable you to attain the success you seek." You have determined to change your way of thinking, and that determination is now driving your commitment to take action.

That commitment to take action brings me to my second point: the courage of commitment requires consistency and persistence. You were so determined to ride that bike so you could hang with your friends that you committed to getting up on it and trying. Persistence and consistency kept you getting back on that bike every time you fell. Consistency is about being disciplined enough to continue to work toward your goal regardless of external forces.

As you work on firing your negative self-talk, you will face a lot of external forces. Unexpected schedule changes are going to pop up and keep you from reading this book when you planned to. When you start cutting people out of your life, they may start exerting pressure on you to distract you from your goals. Staying disciplined, persistent, and consistent is the key!

When you pair consistency with persistence, you can't lose. Persistent people push through setbacks and roadblocks when pursuing a goal. When external forces come your way, acknowledge them but keep moving. Maintain your determination, remain committed, stay consistent, and *endure!*

In his book *On Writing*, the author Stephen King tells a story that illustrates consistency and persistence. King had determined that he wanted to be an author, so he committed to writing. When he was young, he nailed a small nail into his bedroom wall to hang his rejection letters. "By the time I was fourteen, the nail in my wall would no longer support the weight of the rejection slips impaled on it," he wrote. "I replaced the nail with a spike and kept writing." If he hadn't stayed consistent in his writing and persisted despite all those rejection letters, we may never have had all of his celebrated books.

Take control of your thoughts to get what you want out of life. Determine. Commit. Be Consistent. Persist.

> ## During your life, never stop dreaming. No one can take away your dreams.
>
> —TUPAC SHAKUR

Today's Tool

Your tool today is the Dream List you will create in today's workout. Complete your list and frame your plans!

Day 10 Workout: Map Out Your Dream List

For today's workout, you will create a dream board with all your dreams on it. Start by creating a list of dreams and goals you want to reach. This list will help you bring your thoughts together to achieve your goals, dreams, and visions.

Once you have made your list, create a dream board by transferring the items on your list to a board. It's like creating a vision board without cutting out all of the images from a magazine. You can also simply print your list and frame it. I know that dream boards are traditionally done at the beginning of the year, but a reset button can be pushed at any time.

Here is an example of my Personal Dream List 2021.

MY PERSONAL DREAM LIST 20__

1. Envision & list everything that you have ever wanted to do, wanted to go, or place you wanted to live in your life.
2. List the relationships types wanted: Parents, husband, wife, significant other, children, co-worker, etc.
3. List your Career Goal, Business, Investment, Chariable
4. Other: Spiritual, Emotional, Physical, Financial or Experiences

Goals/Dreams/Wants

1. _____

2. _____

3. _____

4. _____

5. _____

6. _____

7. _____

8. _____

9. _____

10. _____

11. _____

12. _____

13. _____

Mirror Self-Admiration Chat

Today, give yourself some self-admiration by saying out loud into the mirror:

I, _____, am so proud of myself for organizing and mapping out my dreams, my goals, and my wants.

Day 10: What an amazing accomplishment. Have a blessed and prosperous day on purpose!

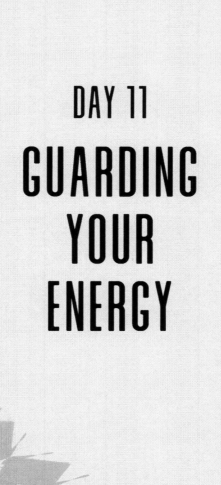

DAY 11
GUARDING YOUR ENERGY

DAY 11

GUARDING YOUR ENERGY

In June 2020 I created a private women's group on Facebook. I refer to the women in this group as my Queen Sisters, and every Wednesday night we have our weekly "Girl Talk Live" time. This group is a safe space that allows the women to choose topics for discussion. I received a message from one of my Queen Sisters asking me to speak on submission. She was concerned about being mistreated in her marriage because her husband was demanding that she be more submissive.

Being a woman in my third marriage, I immediately noticed negative self-talk trying to sneak in. It wasn't something I had said to myself but something that was said to me. In 2014, before I married my current husband, I was having a conversation with a loved one who means the world to me, and she started talking about an issue in her marriage. I assumed that she wanted advice, and attempted to give her my recommendation. However, she wasn't pleased with my opinion and began to attack me by saying, "You aren't qualified to give me advice on my marriage because you have never had a successful marriage! I've been married for ten-plus years!" I hadn't realized how badly her attack hurt me until this topic on submission hit my inbox prior to the group meeting.

Even as a life coach who focuses on eliminating negative self-talk, I was impacted by that particular naysayer all these years later. The good news is that I acknowledged it on the spot instead of using it as an excuse not to help the women who need me most. I had to protect my energy. I had to remember that God allows us to go through life challenges for the experience, in order to help others. I immediately fired the thought that arose— U R FIRED! I FIRED DAT AZZ—and had an amazing chat with the queens that evening.

Be aware of the things that threaten your energy. Negative energy can come from several sources. We all know people whom we dread having to deal with. Watch out for them, and separate yourself, especially if you don't have to have them in your circle.

Our energy can also be affected by the environment we are in. This may be because of the multiple places and people that you associate with, or how the environment is set up; for example, some people are affected by clutter. And then, of course, your negative self-talk affects your energy. One of the major steps along this journey is learning to guard your energy.

This anonymous quote caught my attention on Instagram:

To protect your energy
It's okay to cancel a commitment.
It's okay to not answer that call.
It's okay to change your mind.
It's okay to want to be alone.
It's okay to take a day off.
It's okay to do nothing.
It's okay to speak up.
It's okay to let go.

These points are so true. Preserving your mental and emotional energy is important for your overall health and well-being. Other people's negative energy can cause you to take action that will lead to negative results. If you don't protect your energy, then your energy gas tank will slowly empty—and you can't fuel yourself from an empty tank.

When you have a scheduled meeting with a particular person at work, do you get tense just thinking about what's to come? Whenever a certain family member calls, do you think, *Oh, I don't want to talk to her*? Do you lose sleep thinking about somewhere you have to go? These are triggers—people or things that deplete your energy and often cause you to engage in negative self-talk. We all have them. You need to be aware of your triggers so that you can prepare for, avoid, or set boundaries for your engagement.

Set healthy limits and boundaries to guard your energy. There will be people in your life who will try you; you know, those naysayers who never have anything positive to say and constantly express negative or pessimistic views. There will always be people who say you aren't good enough, you are wasting your time, you can't accomplish this, you will never succeed, I am better than you, you are the weakest link. The important thing is not to accept their ignorance and let it characterize who you are.

It might be necessary for you to control how much time you spend listening to the naysayers. Set clear limits and boundaries with people, nicely cutting them off at the pass if they get critical or mean. Remember, "no" is a complete sentence. It's okay to not answer the phone. It's okay to cancel a commitment because you aren't feeling up to dealing with the naysayer. When you do have to deal with the naysayers, don't allow them to define you. Redirect the conversation toward a more positive discussion. Detach yourself from their negative emotions. The ultimate goal is your well-being, not them and the stupid stuff they have to say!

The harmful things that others say can cut you deep. The pain feels like it goes all the way down to your soul. But that doesn't mean that the fight is over or you can't succeed. Giving up should not be an option. You have to refuse to go down without a fight. Keep pushing to build your thought progression. Your happiness depends on it.

If I had listened to the naysayers, I would still be in the Austrian Alps yodeling.

—ARNOLD SCHWARZENEGGER

Today's Tool

Sometimes when we're triggered or have to deal with naysayers, we get anxious, which then affects our ability to make decisions that are in our best interests and to fire that negative self-talk. There are a lot of tools to help you with anxiety; I recommend a breathing app called Awesome Breathing, described as a "pacer for meditation and stress," by Awesome Labs LLC. It is free on both Androids and iPhones. Use this amazing app daily to help with meditation, sleep, stress, anxiety, or to help bring calmness to your day and restore your energy.

Day 11 Workout: Fire the Naysayers

Today I want you to do a little reminiscing on things that others have told you that you couldn't succeed in, and then you are going to FIRE DAT AZZ! Steve Harvey talks about how his sixth-grade teacher told him that he would never be on television. Look at him now!

Here are a couple of examples to get you started. Add any of your own that come to mind:

_____ told me that I couldn't _____. I FIRED DAT AZZ and know that I can do anything I want to do.

_____ told me that I'd never amount to anything. I FIRED DAT AZZ and know that I am enough and I am somebody.

Mirror Self-Admiration Chat

Today, give yourself some self-admiration by saying out loud into the mirror:

I, _____, am so proud of myself for not allowing naysayers to define who I become.

Day 11: What an amazing accomplishment. Have a blessed and prosperous day on purpose!

DAY 12

SELF-REFLECTION
#2

DAY 12

SELF-REFLECTION #2

It's time for another self-reflection day to see and appreciate your progress. I want you to digest everything you have learned about yourself so far, and just love on yourself! This is also a great time to catch up or go back and read over some previous days that impacted you the most.

> We do not learn from experience;
> we learn from reflecting on experience.
>
> —JOHN DEWEY

Today's Tool

An accountability partner is an awesome tool, and is even more valuable if you choose a life coach as your partner. Before you start with any coach, be sure to verify that the coach is a good fit for you and your goals. The value lies in your success when you invest in yourself.

An accountability partner can be helpful in many areas of your life:

- ➲ They are inspirational and motivational.
- ➲ The can help you commit to tasks and goals.
- ➲ They are your support person.
- ➲ They can help you to stay focused.
- ➲ They can help you to build momentum.

Day 12 Workout: Self-Reflection #2

Today is the time to reflect on how you have progressed in all of the strengths you have developed so far, and how much you have gained control over your negative self-talk.

Questionnaire

Rate your progress after participating in days 1 through 11 using the scale below. Make a note of the points you give each question, then add them up at the end.

never (0 pts) sometimes (1 pt) above average (2 pts) most of the time (3 pts) all of the time (5 pts)

1) I am fully committed and staying consistent in my self-talk journey.

2) I have been able to acknowledge and evaluate my self-talk daily.

3) I have consistently fired my negative self-talk throughout this journey.

4) I am still pinpointing areas that my negative thoughts stem from.

5) I am able to recognize the areas where I am self-sabotaging.

6) Retraining my mind is working for me.

7) I am excited to learn more.

TOTAL: _____

0 pts = no progress
1 to 7 pts = very little progress
8 to 14 pts = some progress (recommend you reread days 1 through 5)
15 to 21 pts = moving in the right direction
22 to 28 pts = amazing job
29 to 35 pts = You are 100 percent ready for the next step in your journey.

Day 12 Bonus Workout

Today you get a second bonus workout identical to Day 6! In the space provided, write some notes and thoughts that support your self-reflection and self-love.

Notes to Self:

Mirror Self-Admiration Chat

Today, give yourself some self-admiration by saying out loud into the mirror:

I, _____, am so proud of myself for loving myself unconditionally.

Day 12: What an amazing accomplishment. Have a blessed and prosperous day on purpose!

DAY 13

MEASURING YOUR GROWTH

DAY 13

MEASURING YOUR GROWTH

I really wanted to write this book, but I struggled! My negative self-talk told me I didn't have time, so I started by trying to delegate and hire someone else to do it. My naysayer said that I wasn't good enough. My writing wasn't clear or understandable. Too many people have already written on this topic. I was even told that I wasn't a good fit for them to help me! But as you can see, I didn't give up.

To overcome this challenge, I first identified what the problem was: it was me! I had a deadline in mind, but I kept making the excuse that I didn't have time to get things done for the book because I had other things to do. It wasn't that I didn't have enough time; it was that I had not dedicated time to complete my book because my self-talk told me that since I had never done it, I couldn't do it. As far as the naysayers, they were irrelevant.

Once I identified the problem, I then had to determine whether it was a reason or an excuse. This is a serious area that is easy to be in denial about. I've worked with hundreds of clients who have long lists of "reasons" why they can't make their goals. These are actually excuses that they sincerely believe are reasons to not succeed. Reasons are not controllable; you have no control over them. Excuses are controllable. Making time to devote to my book was controllable; therefore, I was using an excuse to avoid working on my book.

Of course, I overcame that excuse by choosing to FIRE DAT AZZ! I said to myself, *Samantha, you know that's not a reason. That is a flat-out excuse!* In order to grow, we have to call ourselves out when necessary. Once I fired that negative self-talk and those excuses, I had to figure out a solution. This is where we get to the meat of this improvement plan. I had to figure out how to overcome the excuse that I had created of not having enough time. I developed an active improvement plan that helped me to self-reflect.

Here's my active improvement plan:

Use my improvement plan as a guide for you to create your own plan:

I want to improve on the time I dedicate to my book project. Between managing my group and trying to create content for my group members, I realized that I have not allocated equal time to outlining my book and beginning my writing process. After speaking with my editor I realized that the work is already there. I just have to put the ideas in book form.

THE PLAN
- Gather all notes from sessions
- Organize notes by outlined chapters
- Highlight key topics
- Create sub-topics
- Work on conclusion
- Gather all social media links
- Resource materials

Your Improvement Plan

Your improvement plan will look different from mine. The goal is to have a plan that allows you to acknowledge the negative self-talk, overcome it, and find ways to succeed at whatever you want to do. This written document will show you how great you are at overcoming problems, and also serves as a useful guide forward.

I also use my active improvement plan as a form of self-reflection. I develop a plan for how to reach my current goal, thinking through all of the negative self-talk that could get in my way. This helps me to get my thoughts and decisions in order and to notice patterns to my behavior and thoughts.

I love the quote, "What gets measured, improves." Although it is typically used when referring to business initiatives, it can just as easily be applied to our personal lives. I'm not talking about measurement in its literal sense; I'm talking about reflection. You just finished a day of reflection in Day 12. Hopefully, you reflected on how you felt and who you were at the beginning of this journey, and on changes you have made along the way. Reflecting on how you feel now and other goals you want to reach is also beneficial.

Self-reflection is important to measuring your growth. It will help you to sit with yourself and analyze what you have done, why you have done it, how you have changed, and the tools you used to change. This self-reflection helps you to focus on what is going on within you, which then helps you to identify triggers, self-sabotage, and all of the little ways that other people, and we ourselves, get in the way of our progress. Recall John Dewey's quote, that we don't learn from experience; we learn from reflecting on experience. Make self-reflection a regular part of your life, even after you finish this journey.

One method of self-reflection and measuring your growth is journaling. In an interview, Kelly Rowland said that journaling was her method of self-reflection because recording the details of what she had gone through allowed her to look back and see how far she had come. But I think what was really important about what she said was that journaling made her proud to see her progress and how she made it through a bad situation. Can you imagine the impact that can have on your negative self-talk!!??!! To see, in your own words and handwriting, the discipline you exercised to achieve great things. Reading your own success will have you FIRING DAT AZZ real fast!

Meditation is a wonderful method of self-reflection—and don't go there with the I-can't-quiet-my-mind excuse. When I say meditation, I mean taking the time to look inward and see what thoughts arise. You can meditate while sitting, strolling through a garden, and even going on a run. The key is just to be with yourself and observe whatever thoughts arise, then think about those thoughts and consider how they relate to your growth.

Your vision will become clear only when you can look into your own heart. Who looks outside, dreams; who looks inside, awakes.

—CARL JUNG

Today's Tool

Continue to use your apps to stay focused, inspired, and consistent. And now, clear your mind, because you are going to put all the pieces of your journey together.

Day 13 Workout: Vision Board

My Queen Sister, we have covered a lot today! And it was all necessary. As today's workout quote by Carl Jung says, you have to self-reflect in order for your visions to become clear, and I want you to achieve the visions you have for your future.

This week's workout is developing a vision board, a fun tool to help you clarify and maintain your focus on what truly matters to you. You can use your Dream List from Day 10 or you start something from scratch to guide you. If you're really ambitious, think about which visions you can apply an improvement plan to after you develop your vision board.

It is important that you ask yourself specific questions to inspire you while creating your vision board, because what you put on your vision board will represent what you want to bring into your life. Carefully choose images that are meaningful to you. The goal is to create a visual representation of your goals and dreams to help you stay focused and inspired. Here are some questions to ask yourself:

- ➲ What do I want my life to look like?
- ➲ What does success look like to me?
- ➲ What does my family time look like to me?
- ➲ How do I want to serve others?

Here is an example of my vision board.

Figure 3. Samantha's Vision Board

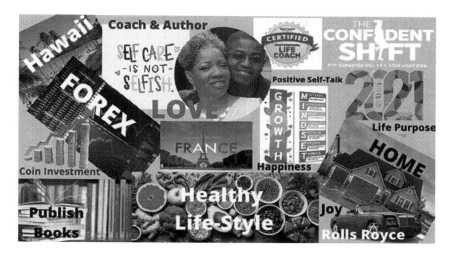

Create Your Vision Board Here

Mirror Self-Admiration Chat

Today, give yourself some self-admiration by saying out loud into the mirror:

I, _____ am so proud of myself for making continual progress and improvement.

Day 13: What an amazing accomplishment. Have a blessed and prosperous day on purpose!

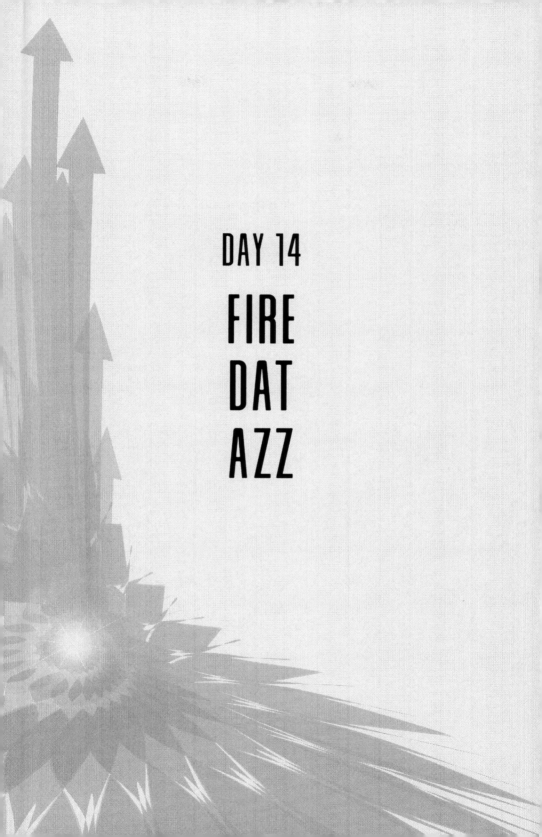

DAY 14

FIRE
DAT
AZZ

FIRE DAT AZZ

"What's going on? Why am I being called to the HR office?" asked Betty. She knew that she hadn't met the required productivity, but she dreaded getting terminated even if she did hate the job. She never gave her all. She preferred to distract herself by socializing with other unproductive employees instead of focusing on her daily tasks. She went into the office with her usual unpleasant attitude.

Betty wasn't pleased when the HR manager began to go over her termination paperwork. The manager explained to her that the company follows a point system, which was in the job description when Betty was hired. He presented her with her production progress form, her warning write-ups, and her performance review sheets, all of which she had signed. Finally, he said, "Here is your signed agreement listing your responsibilities. You have not been able to meet these requirements or the company's expectations. This opportunity is no longer working as a result of your underperformance. Unfortunately, you are not a good fit for this position."

Have you ever been fired before? One of the steps that occurs before being terminated is a one-on-one talk with your boss. They usually bring you into the office to discuss work-related issues. Maybe you were late for work one too many times, and they could no longer look past it. Perhaps you didn't meet your goals and were no longer a good fit for the position. Whatever the reason, it was time to have the hard conversation that no one wants to have. You were about to be terminated. Your boss knew it, and deep down, you did, too. You had that gut feeling, the one where your heart feels like it has sunk into your stomach, the feelings of nausea and fear because you didn't know what would happen next—let's keep those feelings right where they are.

Now visualize that YOU are that boss and your negative thoughts are the employees. I have provided you with all the skills you need to manage those "employees" right out the door! It is time to do some restructuring of your entire "company" (mindset).

Acknowledging the negative self-talk, analyzing your origin story, and recognizing self-sabotage has helped you to see that these "employees" aren't contributing to the good of the organization and that they are poor performers. You have gained the courage necessary to make a change, and have done the work to retrain your mind. Looking back, you can see that you have come a long way, and now it's time for you to FIRE those negative thoughts once and for all.

Now I want you to adopt a boss behavior with the tools you have learned to do so. On previous days you acknowledged that you have negative self-talk and determined where it comes from. You now have many tools to help you eliminate it from your life. Remember, you are the BOSS over your thoughts! You know what is good for your "organization" (you), and you have control over everything. Repeat after me: "I control my thoughts; my thoughts do not control me!"

Now, whenever you have thoughts of "I'm not good enough," or "I don't know how I'll get this done because I am not good at," I want you to stop, remember that you are the top BOSS, and then FIRE DAT AZZ!

Say it with me: U R FIRED! I FIRED DAT AZZ!

LOUDER: "U R FIRED! I FIRED DAT AZZ!"

Terminate your negative self-talk by FIRING DAT AZZ!

—SAMANTHA HILL

Today's Tool

Today's tool is a letter of termination. You will be drafting this letter to forever FIRE the negative self-talk. This self-talk has broken all the rules, and you will no longer accept this behavior. It's time to totally commit to releasing that negative self-talk.

You can follow this template or make your own:

Termination Letter to Negative Self-Talk

SUBJECT: Termination of Service

Dear Ms. Negative Self-Talk Thinker,

In our previous one-on-one sessions, you were advised to give more attention to your duties and improve your performance. However, no improvement has been seen. You are affecting the progress and growth of _____.

Therefore, I am excited to inform you that on behalf of the CEO, U R FIRE

D! Your services have been terminated immediately and without pay. You may obtain your permanent clearance certificate, titled U R FIRED! I FIRED DAT AZZ!, on your way out of my brain.

I wish you the best in never entering anyone's brain again.

Yours sincerely,

_____

CEO/BOSS Over My Thoughts

Now write your own letter of termination:

Day 14 Workout: Hang Your Letter of Termination

Once you have perfected your letter of termination, it's time to hang it proudly for all negative "employees" to see. Today's workout will bring your letter of Termination to life.

Step 1: Print, sign, and frame your Letter of Termination. Hang it where you can see it daily as a reminder of your commitment to continue to FIRE DAT AZZ whenever negative self-talk attempts to show itself.

Step 2: Record yourself on your electronic device reading your letter of termination with confidence. This way, you can listen to or watch it any time you feel your negative self-talk sneaking into your thoughts. Stay consistent, and don't look back.

Mirror Self-Admiration Chat

Today, give yourself some self-admiration by saying out loud into the mirror:

I, _____, am so proud of myself for terminating my negative self-talk daily.

Day 14: What an amazing accomplishment. Have a blessed and prosperous day on purpose!

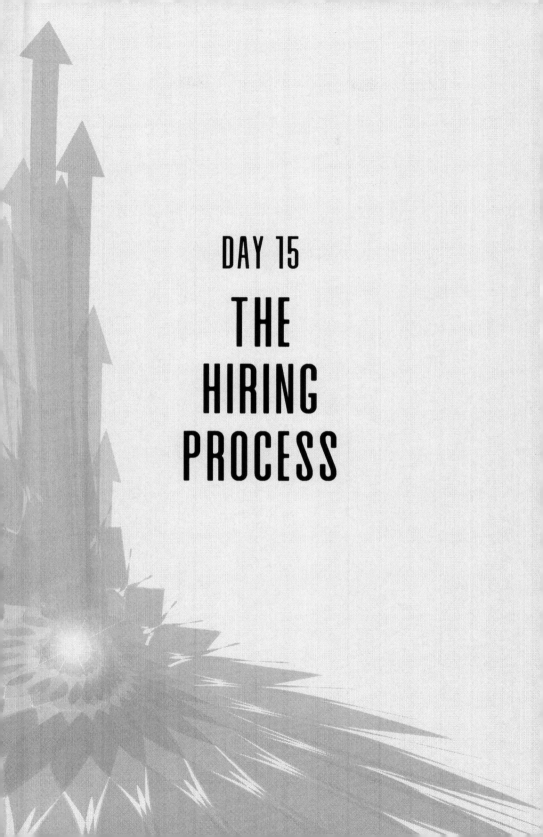

DAY 15
THE HIRING PROCESS

DAY 15

THE HIRING PROCESS

Once I finally had my lightbulb moment of seeing that celebrities focus on being the best in their field, I felt as if I had denied myself the ultimate type of love for so many years. It was unintentional, but it had negatively impacted my self-talk. Like so many others, I had wanted to be loved since my early childhood.

I remember crying in my old, antique-style bottom bunk bed because I wanted that motherly love but didn't get it. How do you feel loved without receiving hugs or being told that you are loved? I went through my two divorces because I didn't feel loved. How could I after being manipulated, beaten, and cheated on? I didn't feel loved by friends and family. How could I after being cussed out, lied to, and talked about? My search for love wasn't pleasant.

Over my lifetime, I have craved love from my mother, father, children, friends, family, teachers, and the world, to love me for being me. Thank God I have grown and now understand where true love lies; I now realize that the most important love is self-love. My self-love allowed me to develop the positive self-talk that I now give myself. Once I created the ultimate self-love within myself, I grew into a different person. Along the way, I lost many people who I thought would be beside me for life. However, I have gained a lot of strong, loving, like-minded people throughout my new journey.

Research has proven that positive thinking lowers the risk of cancer and has many other benefits, including:

- ⮑ reduced stress
- ⮑ better sleeping habits
- ⮑ longer life span
- ⮑ healthier body
- ⮑ protection against lung disease
- ⮑ reduced chance of heart disease and stroke

Let's decide together to let go of the past hurts, negativities, and thoughts. It has never helped us in any degree to prosper in life. I am truly proud of you and the journey you have taken. You have set yourself on a path to a more fruitful way of thinking by hiring a more positive YOU.

You made a COMMITMENT TO SELF at the beginning of this journey, and we have touched on a host of ways you can incorporate the firing process in your daily routine. Today you will write a PROMISE TO SELF letter to seal the deal on your positive thinking by using the hiring process. The purpose of this letter is to help you to become a more optimistic and positive person by continually committing to your ultimate goal for life, and to live a longer, happier, and healthy life.

This "hiring process" consists of focusing on thoughts with certain qualities, positive self-talk, and consciously bringing joy and happiness into your mind. The following table compares hiring an employee for a job and hiring positive thoughts for life.

Table 1. The Hiring Process

HIRING AN EMPLOYEE	HIRING POSITIVE THOUGHTS
Permanent long-term employee	Permanent long-term thoughts
Action-taker with growth potential	Action-taker with growth potential
Problem solver in difficult situation	Problem solver in difficult situation
Dedicated, with positive personality	Dedicated, with positive personality

As you can see, hiring a new employee and hiring positive thoughts are the same concept. Creating the hiring strategy for your mindset will include a positive thinking approach to receive that positive outcome that you desire. Positive thinking makes positive things happen for better results in your daily journey. To start the process of strengthening your mindset, here are some things to be mindful of throughout your journey:

> Don't be hard on yourself. You will make mistakes, and negative self-talk will sneak in from time to time. You are human. Just push your reset button and start again by hiring new positive thoughts.

> Be accountable so that you will correct yourself. Connect with an accountability partner/coach for support. Hire the thought, "I messed up, but I got this."

> Celebrate your accomplishment daily. Be proud of yourself, and accept other people's compliments. Don't hire any "yeah but" or "I'm not" thoughts.

> Interview and acknowledge your thoughts.

It is important to continue to control your negative self-talk. Promise yourself to fight for a happier and healthier life. You can't control everything; however, you can promise to never give up. Know that you deserve the best. Positive people produce great role models, challenge their thoughts, and focus on solutions instead of problems. Positive people also have a great impact on other people.

The most important person to keep your promise to is yourself.

Today's Tool

Today's tool will mark the completion of your journey through 15 days of firing negative self-talk and hiring positive thoughts. Today you will write a promise to yourself to hire positive self-talk, celebrate yourself, and commit once again to be the boss over your thoughts. Here is a sample letter you can use, or create your own.

My Promise to Self Letter

I, _____, promise to continue taking action to strengthen and build my inner thoughts in a positive manner, just as I committed to at the beginning of my journey.

Even though I have spent my entire life indulging in negative self-talk, I promise to challenge my thoughts from now on. I promise to hold myself accountable and to stay consistent.

I promise to celebrate myself and to create a weekly healthy self-love and self-care routine. I promise to remember that self-love is one of the greatest gifts to reward myself with.

I promise to always practice being the boss over my thoughts.

I promise to stay on top of my thoughts and to never allow them to drag me down. I promise to remove the words "I can't," "I hate," "I'm not good enough," "I'm not good at," "I want to, but," "what if," "it's too late," and "I'm too old" from my self-talk.

I will always do my best to uphold these commitments to myself by repeatedly saying the following affirmations daily:

I AM ENOUGH.
I AM WORTHY.

Signed _____
Date _____

Use this space to write your own version of the letter.

Day 15 Workout: Complete Your Journey

For your workout today, you will make your letter a reality. Follow these instructions:

Step 1: Print, sign, and frame your Promise to Self Letter. Hang it where you can see it daily as a reminder of your promise to continue the hiring process after firing the negative self-talk.

Step 2: Record yourself on your electronic device reading your promise to self letter with confidence. This way you can listen to or watch it at any time.

Mirror Self-Admiration Chat

Today, give yourself some self-admiration by saying out loud into the mirror:

I, _____, am so proud of myself for promising to love myself and be the BOSS over my thoughts.

Day 15: What an amazing accomplishment. Have a blessed and prosperous day on purpose!

THE WRAP-UP

This journey has been teaching you to know that you are a boss, the ruler over your own thoughts, and how to fire your negative thinking through the fire/hire process.

We have focused on becoming a more positive thinker, building a better you, and acknowledging your control over your thoughts. Continue to build positive thinking into your life daily. Here are some positive affirmations that you can repeat daily:

I control my thoughts; my thoughts do not control me.

I am in control of my happiness today, tomorrow, and into the future.

I commit to challenging myself to grow daily.

I say 'YES' to my joy.

I challenge you to use all of the information I have shared on this journey create a better version of yourself, and I encourage you to share these tips with others. Should you ever find yourself in a place where you think you are not strong enough to press forward, reach out and take your personal journey again by reading this book as many times as needed. I also encourage you to join our amazing Facebook group of Queen Sisters, and become part of a large group of women who began their journey just as you did. None of us truly comes into this journey knowing where we will end up. Starting is the key!

Continue to journal your thoughts to keep track of your progress. Revisit the affirmations you set for yourself. Surround yourself with people who speak positive things about you, to you, and with you. Your environment is so important. Terminate anything that makes you feel like you are incapable of being better. Any time you feel like you will slip back into those old thoughts you have worked so hard to overcome, remember to say these words: U R FIRED! I FIRED DAT AZZ!

YOU MADE IT! It's time for your final celebration, my Queen Sister. This is the moment you have been waiting for. You have been longing to get to this point from the moment you opened this book. Congratulate yourself! Give yourself a pat on the back and a huge hug. Treat yourself out to a day on the town. Tell yourself how proud you are for overcoming some of the biggest hurdles in your life by firing your self-talk, removing the excuses, reducing your fears, and eliminating your self-doubt.

A prepared destiny awaits you. Your actions through this journey have groomed you for a successful future in self-love. My purpose in writing this book is not to rush you through the process of terminating negative self-talk but to guide you, step-by-step, through each stage at your own pace. I pray that you will see all of the manifestations and blessings that you deserve.

But this is not the end. I want you to recognize that the life you live, that you have planned for, and that you may hope for can become reality with discipline. You have to be disciplined enough to hold yourself accountable for where you want to be, what you say, how you act, and how you project your energy onto others. Such discipline requires action every day.

As you have learned, much of our toxic behavior stems from years of hearing the same negative words from those whom we love and care about. Our families, friends, colleagues, and others project their fears, negative self-talk, and inferiority onto us, and we often mirror those same behaviors. What you have learned over the years cannot be changed in fifteen days.

Carry this book with you, mark the pages that resonate with you, and highlight sections to refer back to. The message here is to prepare yourself to complete any task you desire and reach any goal without self-sabotaging your joy and happiness. It's time for you to mirror the positive attributes we have discussed so that you can be a reflection of those same things to others.

I desire to create a legacy for all the Queen Sisters who adopt positive self-talk, positive thoughts, inspiring ideas, and do the work behind those things for continuous growth.

As a final reflection, I want you to list two or three people whom you feel can benefit from this book, and why. Be detailed in your response. Part of your mission will be to touch the lives of others, as this book has done for you. Whether you work in a corporate setting or are an educator, business owner, or a stay-at-home mom, you have a responsibility to serve those around you, and you can only do that if you are being your best self.

What an amazing accomplishment. Have a blessed and prosperous day on purpose!

Final Notes to Self:

ABOUT THE AUTHOR

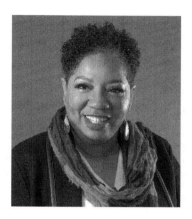

Samantha Wisdom Hill is a southern girl from Jackson, Mississippi, where she worked as a licensed cosmetologist. When she was in elementary school, she started braiding her neighbors' hair on her mom's front porch for two dollars a head. Looking back, she realizes she was already developing her coaching skills at that time.

Samantha earned an Associate's degree in Applied Science and a Bachelor of Business Administration degree in Management. She is also a certified nutritional microscopist trained in using living food as nutritional medicine and microscopic live blood analysis of enzyme potential.

Her passion and true focus is as a Certified Master Life Coach who helps women to shift their negative self-talk, find their confidence, true voice, and regain their power through her coaching and her new book, *Shift Your Confidence*!

She desires to use her voice to encourage and empower women so she does not have to watch another woman die without finding her joy in her lifetime. She has seen so many women just give up and accept their painful life cycle as the cards that they were dealt, believing that it's too late to change the life they created.

Samantha is blessed to be a wife, the mother of four children and a stepson, and grandmother of three grandsons. As a spiritual woman, Samantha's greatest purpose is to use her voice however God says to use it. When all has been said and done, her ultimate goal is for God to say, "Servant, well done!"

Currently, she works with small groups and with one-on-one clients, helping them to find confidence and live a life of happiness by achieving their goals and their purpose in life. Samantha encourages women to be the boss over their thoughts instead of accepting whatever life throws them.

Join her Private Facebook Group: https://www.facebook.com/groups/confidenceforwomenwithsamantha

Learn more about Samantha: http://confidentshift.com.

Made in the USA
Coppell, TX
11 February 2022

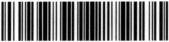